H. PYLORI
Rescue Guide

Written by:		Photography:		Art director:
Angela Privin		**Angela Privin**		**Beatriz Abreu**

CONTENT

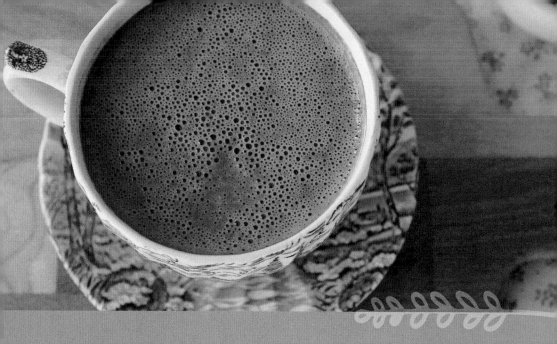

H. PYLORI RESCUE GUIDE

I am a health coach and not a doctor, so nothing in this guide is to be taken as medical advice. This material is for educational purposes only. Always check with your doctor for counter indications/interference with current medications before starting any new supplements.

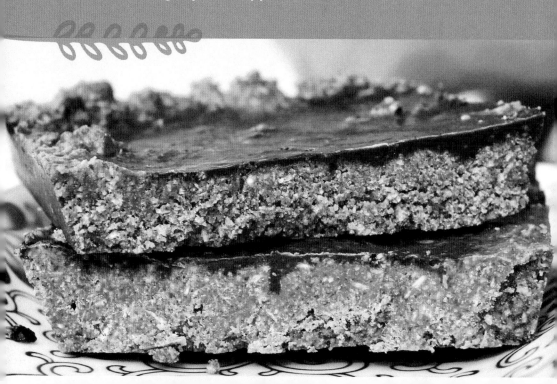

H. PYLORI RESCUE

H. pylori is a spiral-shaped bacteria that infects the stomach, lowers stomach acid and compromises digestion. It lives in the stomach's mucosal layer and can damage and inflame the stomach lining.

When h. pylori overgrows it can cause digestive symptoms like bloating, gas, burping, pain, nausea, constipation and reflux. It can also cause fatigue, anxiety and depression in some people.

H. pylori lowers stomach acid in most people, which compromises the digestion of all food, particularly meat, beans, complex grains and raw veggies.

Stomach acid also protects from pathogens by killing them before they enter the small intestine. Low stomach acid compromises this built-in protection and leaves the body vulnerable to infections.

H. pylori can damage the gut through the downstream effect it has on the biome, opening the door to parasitic infections, bacterial imbalance and yeast overgrowth.

For this reason, h. pylori is often the root cause AND missing piece for fixing difficult or unresponsive digestive problems.

Because h. pylori is a gateway infection, it should be addressed first, and will dramatically improve the chances of clearing other gut infections.

Eradicating h. pylori can help stomach acid bounce back, finally giving the gut an opportunity to heal, rebalance and repair.

I wrote this guide for people who test positive for h. pylori and don't know what it is or what to do about it.

Antibiotics are not the best solution because this infection is becoming increasingly harder to kill due to antibiotic overuse and resistance as well as biofilms barriers.

H. pylori can be fixed naturally if it is addressed correctly. I will teach you how to do this right so it's not stubborn to eradicate or has a low likelihood of returning.

And if natural herbs don't eradicate the infection in the first round due to severity, they won't damage the biome like antibiotics can.

I've worked with many clients with h. pylori in my health coaching practice and have had it myself, so this guide is based on extensive research and experience.

HISTORY OF H. PYLORI

Helicobacter pylori was discovered in 1982 by two Australian scientists, Robin Warren and Barry J. Marshall as a causative factor for ulcers.

In their original paper, Warren and Marshall contended that most stomach ulcers and gastritis were caused by colonization with this bacteria, and not just by stress or spicy food as was assumed before.

The h. pylori hypothesis was poorly received, so in an act of self-experimentation Marshall drank a culture of h. pylori bacteria extracted from a patient and five days later developed gastritis.

His symptoms disappeared after two weeks, but he took antibiotics to kill the remaining bacteria. This experiment was published in 1984 in the Australian Medical Journal and remains highly cited.

In 1997, government health agencies, academic institutions, and industry, launched a national education campaign to teach health care providers and patients about the link between h. pylori and ulcers.

Having h. pylori does not mean you will have an ulcer, but it raises your chances of having one.

It's theorized that h. pylori is passed down from a parent to child, spread between spouses or other family members or contracted from contaminated food or water.

It's more common to get h. pylori when living in crowded conditions or traveling to a developing country with less sanitary conditions. But you can get h. pylori anywhere, particularly when your immune defenses are down.

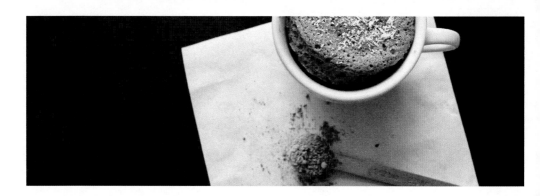

CHALLENGES AND COMMON MISTAKES

The biggest challenges around h. pylori eradication are:

1.-Proper testing

2.- Biofilms

3.-Supporting the adrenals and lowering stress

4.-Bolstering a struggling immune system (SiG A).

Both triple or quadruple antibiotic therapy or natural herbs can fail to eradicate h. pylori if the above factors are not addressed.

In this guide, I will teach you how to navigate these four challenges to increase success rates and avoid common mistakes. Knowing what you are doing will lower stress, which can also increase success.

This guide will also cover how to prevent relapses, minimize transmission and bolster the efficacy of a herbal protocol.

If you've already done a natural protocol with little success, this guide may help fill in the missing pieces. Finding the right dose, doing it for the right length of time, adding a biofilm buster and managing stress can make all the difference.

TESTING FOR H. PYLORI

While there's many ways to do it, h. pylori is hard to test for because it doesn't always show up.

Standard medical testing at the doctor's office, such as the breath test, blood test, stool test and endoscopic biopsy, can fail to identify an active and damaging infection.

These tests are simply not sensitive enough to pick up every overgrowth, so there's a possibility of a false negative.

Functional stool testing is much more sensitive as it uses PCR technology that looks for DNA clues of infection. The test most likely to find h. pylori is the GI Map.

Even on the GI Map, an h. pylori infection can hide. A trained practitioner can spot the classic bacterial patterns that suggests h. pylori is present but hiding.

Here are some clues that suggest h. pylori may be in hiding:

Parasites like dientamoeba fragilis and blastocystis hominis

Candida overgrowth

SIBO (small intestinal bacterial overgrowth)

General overgrowth of bacteria in the large intestine, with a focus on these particular bacterial strains: Akkermansia, pseudomonas, clostridia, klebsiella, morganella, strep and staph.

Low elastase (digestive enzyme production).

These clues are combined with symptoms to identify a hidden infection:

Anxiety, depression, fatigue

Nutritional deficiencies in iron, magnesium, vitamin A, C, E, folic acid and B12.
Ulcers, gastritis, silent reflux (LPR) and acid reflux

Silent reflux is felt as irritation in the larynx, throat and voice box, excess mucus, lump in the throat, raspy voice or constant throat clearing. Excess mucus is produced by the body as a protection against acid in the esophagus.

Note that symptoms of h. pylori can mimic the symptoms of bacterial overgrowth in the small intestine (SIBO) as both can cause bloating, gas, nausea, constipation and reflux.

After some healing and repair work is done on the gut, h. pylori typically shows up on a GI Map retest. When it finally shows on the test it means it has risen to the surface of the mucus lining or the biofilm has broken. Then it becomes easier to kill.

The GI Map is an at home stool test that's used by naturopaths and functional medicine practitioners like myself. If you need help ordering the GI anywhere in the world, contact me through my website at www. diyhealthblog.com

VIRULENT STRAINS OF H. PYLORI

There are many different bacterial strains of h. pylori and some strains can do more damage than others.

The GI Map tests for these damaging, virulent strains of h. pylori. Some virulent strains can increase the occurrence of ulcers and others

bolster chances of gastric cancer. Virulent strains are treated in the same way as less harmful strains. I always suggest addressing h. pylori if it is virulent.

WHY DOES H. PYLORI AFFECT SOME PEOPLE BUT NOT OTHERS?

H. pylori is a common infection that can cause severe symptoms in some people and no symptoms in others.

There is a complex relationship between h. pylori and the host's immune system that balances the bacterial overgrowth and keeps pathogenic effects at bay. Some people do not experience big stomach acid fluctuations with h. pylori, and it does not have a detrimental effect on the biome.

Not everyone with h. pylori needs to be treated, but those who have digestive symptoms, mood issues, nutritional deficiencies or fatigue are likely to benefit from eradication.

People free from issues with digestion, fatigue, body pain, brain fog and mood may have a neutral or even helpful strain of h. pylori. And the overgrowth is likely controlled by the body.

Chronic stress or immune system suppression could turn a neutral infection into a pathogenic one. That is why someone can have h. pylori for a long time, but only start having symptoms after going through a difficult, stressful or hectic period in life.

Running a stool analysis, like the GI Map, provides a comprehensive look at the effects h. pylori is having on the gut and microbiome. And will provide good information about whether or not it should be addressed.

If h. pylori is the root cause of other pathogens in the gut, it should be addressed before tackling the other issues.

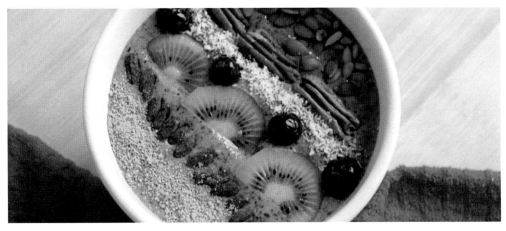

DIFFERENCE BETWEEN H. PYLORI PROTOCOLS

H. pylori can be addressed with either prescription or herbal antibiotics.

Antibiotic therapy is a shorter treatment than herbal intervention and may be covered by insurance. The efficacy of antibiotic therapy was estimated to be between 70 and 80 percent 13 years ago and is declining with time.

But, antibiotics for h. pylori could also damage the biome and create further digestive issues. If the biome is already out of balance, the damage done by antibiotics can be more severe.

You can mitigate antibiotic damage by taking a probiotic supplement called Saccharomyces boulardii, before, during and after treatment.

Also, acid lowering medications are often prescribed with antibiotics. If stomach acid is low, lowering it further can be problematic.

Antibiotic resistance and/or failure to breakdown protective biofilms are reasons why antibiotics can fail.

A natural herbal protocol will take 2 months and must be done at proper therapeutic doses to be effective.

If done correctly, the herbal protocol is very effective, but I advise clinical supervision during your program.

Also, knowing how to troubleshoot roadblocks will up your success rate tremendously. In the next few sections we'll address roadblocks like biofilms, stress and immune status.

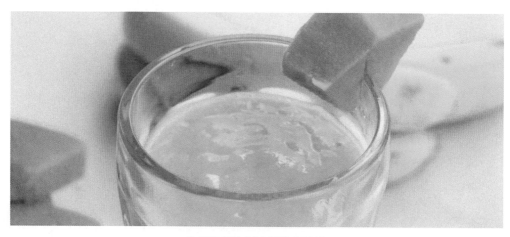

STRESS, ADRENALS AND H. PYLORI

Stress can leave you vulnerable to contracting h. pylori in the first place or cause a relapse. Stress also greatly increases h. pylori levels and worsens symptoms.

Chronic stress can cause h. pylori to morph from a neutral organism to a pathogenic one.

Stress also makes it harder to clear h. pylori.

Some people need to reduce stress and support the adrenals before starting an h. pylori protocol.

You can measure adrenal status with an adrenal cortisol test that takes 3 to 4 cortisol snapshots throughout the day. You can use the Dutch test hormone panel or a simple salivary cortisol test will do.

If the adrenals are depleted, it could take 4 to 8 weeks to recover them. Recovery includes rest, good sleep, balancing blood sugar, taking adaptogenic herbs and lowering stress. My favorite adrenal adaptogen supplement is called Daily Stress Formula by Pure Encapsulations.

This mayo clinic study showed that working on stress and adrenal support alone can lower and improve levels of h. pylori.

IMMUNE SYSTEM AND H. PYLORI

Medicine alone won't do the job. Both herbs and pharmaceuticals partner with the immune system to win the battle against h. pylori.

Strong immune function is crucial to the success of any h. pylori protocol. If the immune system is suppressed it will need to be supported for at least a month before starting eradication.

Gut immunity is measured through a marker called Secretory IgA or sIgA. The GI Map tests this marker.

If sIgA is below 500, immune support is suggested to help win the fight.

If sIgA is below 150, immune support is required and should be done for six weeks prior to starting h. pylori eradication.

The six week immune support protocol consists of herbs and lifestyle changes that lower stress.

The two supplements I use to bolster immunity are Saccharomyces and Immunoglobulins. My favorite brand of immunoglobulins are MegaIgG2000 by Microbiome labs.

With clients, I use two capsules of Saccharomyces boulardii (Sac B) once a day on an empty stomach and an hour away from other supplements. Not only does this yeast-based probiotic support immunity, it also helps clear h. pylori and can be taken during treatment. It is also helpful for candida overgrowth.

Sac B also flushes out a bacteria called clostridia that often overgrows with h. pylori. In some people, clostridia can cause anxiety, obsessive compulsive behavior or trouble sleeping.

I also use four daily capsules of Mega IgG 2000 with clients (can be taken with or without food).

Adrenal supplementation can also help if fatigue is an issue.

BIOFILMS AND HOW TO BUST THEM

Biofilms can protect h. pylori from antimicrobial and immune attack. That's why using a biofilm busting herb can make a big difference.

Biofilms are defensive shields that many bacterial and yeast species build to protect themselves.

Biofilms need to be broken to expose the whole bacterial community to attack.

Not only do biofilms protect h. pylori colonies from eradication, they can also influence test results.

For example, someone can show low levels of h. pylori on a test, when actual levels are higher. That's because a majority of the infection is hiding under biofilm and is not shed in the stool.

In some cases, after breaking down the biofilm and treating the infection, numbers can increase on a retest. This means that the infection was hiding behind biofilms and was bigger than first seen. And will require a longer treatment.

People who do herbal protocols, like Matula tea or mastic gum, for only 30 days can break open biofilms and expose the real level infection, but not treat it long enough to kill it.

If levels go up, instead of down, after treating and testing, it's a sign of progress. You just need to keep going with the protocol. Typically two months is enough for most people, but some may need to do an h. pylori protocol for four months.

There are many options for biofilm-busting herbs. I've listed them below. They are equally effective and you only need one.

Choose the one with the benefit that fits your needs.

NAC:

500 mg, one capsule taken two to three times a day with meals. Aside from being a good biofilm buster, this amino acid is a precursor to glutathione, which makes it a powerful liver detoxifier. It also cleans out the lungs.

BOSWELLIA:

One capsule (300 to 500 mg) two to three times a day with food. Boswelia has powerful antiinflammatory properties and is typically used for supporting immune health and easing symptoms of autoimmune disease.

INTERFACE PLUS:

A biofilm-busting enzyme that's my least favorite option because this product is grown on mold. Follow dosage instructions on the bottle.

BIOCIDIN:

While the other biofilm busters come in capsule form, this is a tincture, so it's easy to dose. Five to 10 drops are taken two to three times a day between meals. This has antimicrobial properties to kill yeast and gut bacteria.

STOMACH ACID CONTROVERSY AND TEST

There's a disagreement about if low or high stomach acid is to blame for upper GI symptoms.

Functional medicine practitioners believe that low stomach acid causes upper GI symptoms like GERD, reflux and heartburn.

Reasons for low stomach acid that have nothing to do with h. pylori are stress, eating too many processed carbs, nutrient deficiencies, allergies, and/or excess alcohol consumption.

Western medical practitioners believe that high stomach acid is to blame for upper GI distress and prescribe acid blocking medications. If stomach acid is already low, then acid lowering medications will make the problem worse and impact digestion.

There is an easy way to test your stomach acid production at home. This test is not medically conclusive and doesn't produce a solid diagnosis, but it can give a clue about stomach acid production.

All you need for this test is baking soda (sodium bicarbonate) and water.

Baking soda and stomach acid (hydrochloric acid) create a chemical reaction in your stomach that makes carbon dioxide, a gas which causes burping.

A burp within three minutes of drinking the baking soda solution may indicate an adequate level of stomach acid.

A burp after three minutes (or not at all) may indicate a low level of stomach acid.

HOW TO DO THE BAKING SODA STOMACH ACID TEST

Because many variables can control the outcome, we increase accuracy by taking this test five consecutive mornings and recording the results.

First thing in the morning (before eating or drinking), mix 1/4 teaspoon of baking soda in four ounces of cold water.

Drink the baking soda solution.

Set a timer and see how long it takes to burp. If you have not burped within five minutes, stop timing.

If your stomach is producing adequate amounts of stomach acid, you'll likely burp within two to three minutes. Any burping after three minutes can indicate low stomach acid.

If stomach acid is low from h. pylori, I don't suggest supporting it with hydrochloric acid (HCL) or acid-raising herbs like bitters. HCL can cause or worsen ulcers if the stomach lining is very inflamed.

And raising stomach acid during an h. pylori protocol will make the bacteria harder to kill as they burrow deeper into the stomach lining. Even lemon juice or apple cider vinegar can be iffy.

Once the h. pylori is gone, stomach acid should naturally bounce back but it may take time. Supporting acid with bitters in the interim is ok.

ADDRESSING SYMPTOMS WHILE HEALING

While some people experience no upper GI symptoms with h. pylori, common symptoms are heartburn/reflux/GERD and stomach pain from an ulcer. It can also cause gastritis or inflammation of the stomach lining.

With a hiatal hernia, the mainstream belief is that too much pressure and acid in the stomach can loosen it, allowing acid to escape upwards.

An explanation from the functional medicine perspective is when stomach acid is too low, the lower esophageal sphincter (LES) fails to shut tightly. Sufficient stomach is needed for it to form a tight, protective seal.

Because it takes time for any protocol to work, there are strategies to find relief for these symptoms.

ULCER REPAIR:

One of the best ulcer remedies is DGL licorice powder. I like **Vital Nutrients** DGL powder because it's pure licorice with no added sweeteners. Mix ⅛ teaspoon in a few ounces of water and drink it 10 to 15 minutes before a meal.

Along with repairing the lining of the stomach and intestines, DGL licorice also kills h. pylori.

Other soothing and repairing herbs are l-glutamine powder, collagen powder and zinc carnosine. These are typically well tolerated, but collagen is not suitable for vegetarians or people with histamine intolerance.

Zinc carnosine enhances the stomach's mucosal defenses and mends gastric ulcers. It also supports small intestinal mucosal integrity and inhibits the inflammatory response of h. pylori.

Lastly, marshmallow root, slippery elm and aloe vera juice help repair the lining of the stomach and intestines. These herbs, however, could trigger symptoms in people with small intestinal bacterial overgrowth.

Vitamin U (also known as MMS) supports ulcer repair and is most commonly found in raw cabbage juice, but can also be taken in supplement form.

Vitamin U, is not an actual vitamin. It helps regenerate gastric mucous damaged by h. pylori and is also an antioxidant. It is particularly helpful in the stomach's recovery after damaging exposure to non steroidal antiinflammatory medication (NSAID) like ibuprofen. NSAIDs can cause ulcers in people who are not infected with h. pylori.

GASTRITIS RELIEF:

To tame the inflammation associated with gastritis I recommend curcumin, the anti inflammatory compound found in turmeric. You can always add more turmeric on your food but supplements will provide much higher concentrations of inflammatory support. Meriva is a highly bioavailable curcumin concentrate.

REFLUX, GERD AND HEARTBURN:

Following the GERD/Reflux/Heartburn reducing diet may help reduce symptoms.

Avoid these common reflux triggers:

Acidic foods like citrus (limes, lemons, oranges), vinegar and tomatoes. Apple cider vinegar in small amounts may be tolerated by some people.

Chocolate

Coffee and high doses of caffeine

Fatty and fried foods. Good fats like olive oil, avocado and coconut are ok, but avoid inflammatory vegetable oils like canola, peanut, soy, sunflower and foods fried in them. Choose lean cuts of meat over fatty ones.

Mint and peppermint can relax the LES sphincter and should be avoided

Carbonated beverages

In some cases, garlic and onion can contribute to symptoms.

There is a less restrictive way to approach diet, which requires tracking and measuring daily food intake. This allows more variety but smaller portions of irritating foods.

It's called the Fast Tract Diet and works with "fermentation potential", capping the daily allowance of fermentable foods.

REPAIRING THE STOMACH LINING

After finishing the protocol it's a good idea to repair the stomach lining.

The same herbs used to repair ulcers also soothe and patch inflamed stomach tissue.

Supplements like L-glutamine, zinc l-carnosine, DGL licorice, aloe, slippery elm and marshmallow are great for repair. Follow the dosage guidelines on each bottle. I suggest choosing two herbs from this list.

You may not start feeling better until this repair work is completed.

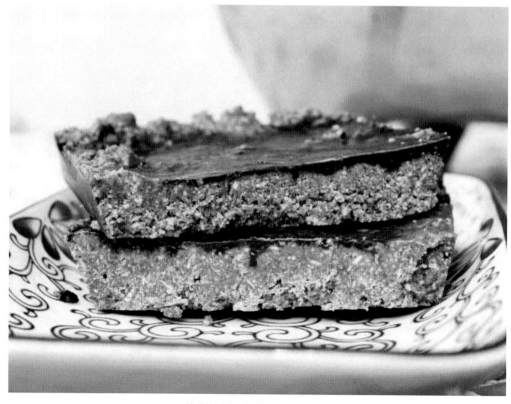

NATURAL PROTOCOLS

Two months is a good length of time to do a protocol. While two months is long enough for most people, aggressive infections may require four months of herbs.

After the first two months, I suggest stopping the protocol, doing some repair work on the stomach lining and waiting 6 to 8 weeks to retest for h. pylori.

If the infection is still present, an additional two months of herbs is needed.

For this protocol to work you only need one killing herbs and a biofilm buster. It is very important to be consistent with the protocol, do it for long enough and keep stress in check.

Begin any protocol slowly and work up to the full dose. For example, start with one matula tea bag a day and add the second after a few days or start with 2 mastic gum capsules and work up to 6 a day based on your body's reaction.

Add in the biofilm buster a few days later. This way if you react to a supplement, staggering them will allow you to identify the problem.

You can also add support herbs to make the protocol more effective. This is a good idea for stubborn infections.

This is a typical protocol:

Matula tea on an empty stomach first thing in the morning and just before bed.

Or

Mastic gum 3 times a day with meals

1 broccoli sprout supplement 30 minutes before lunch and dinner

2 saccharomyces boulardii two hours after lunch

1 NAC with breakfast and lunch

*For stomach pain, ulcer prevention or reflux add DGL licorice 3 times a day 15 minutes before each meal.

NATURAL KILLING HERBS
(THAT TARGET H. PYLORI WITHOUT DISRUPTING THE BIOME)

MATULA TEA:

This tea is made in South Africa from a mix of native antimicrobial herbs.

One box includes 60 tea bags. This tea is expensive but effective and is all you need for 2 months.

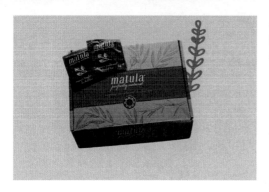

The company guarantees its efficacy. If it doesn't get rid of h. pylori in the first round, they'll refund your money or send you a new package.

My instructions are a bit different from the company's instructions. While they suggest doing the protocol for 30 days and using a fresh tea bag twice a day, I suggest doing it for 60 days and using each tea bag twice (a fresh brew in the morning and reusing the same tea bag at night).

Matula is consumed first thing in the morning and last thing at night on an empty stomach. That means avoiding food 90 minutes before and after consuming it.

It's a pleasant, mild flavored tea but very powerful. It can cause strong die off symptoms (nausea, flu-like symptoms) in the first 10 days.

Matula also combats yeast overgrowth, so if that's an issue, die off can be more intense.

H. pylori can also live in the mouth and dental cavities, so swishing each sip of matula in your mouth for a few seconds can help kill the h. pylori hiding in the mouth.

MASTIC GUM:

This gum is grown on the Greek Island of Chios.

It is taken 3 times daily with meals, 1000 milligrams per dose (2 capsules). Start with one or two capsules a day and build up to 6 a day slowly (adding one or two capsules every 2 to 3 days).

Typically mastic gum is very well tolerated.

Matula tea and Mastic gum are the two primary killing herbs needed to eradicate h. pylori. You only need one or the other. The following herbs can provide extra support to your protocol if you want to boost efficacy, or can be taken as maintenance after the primary killing protocol is done. They are not compulsory but will raise chances of success. In many cases, but not in all cases, the mastic gum or matula tea can do the job alone.

VITAMIN D:

A study showed[1] lower success rates of antibiotic-based eradication of h. pylori in people with low vitamin D levels. This suggests that vitamin D supplementation may increase the chances of protocol success in those who are lacking. 1000 to 5000 IU is a good daily dose depending on level of depletion.

[1]El Shahawy MS, Hemida MH, El Metwaly I, Shady ZM. The effect of vitamin D deficiency on eradication rates of Helicobacter pylori infection. JGH Open. 2018;2(6):270-275. Published 2018 Aug 2. doi:10.1002/jgh3.12081.

After you are finished with your matula tea or mastic gum protocol you can use the supportive herbs below to prevent an h. pylori relapse, particularly during stressful times.

BISMUTH:

This is the active ingredient used in pepto bismol. Don't be alarmed if it turns your poop black.

NIGELLA SATIVA/BLACKSEED OIL:

This is the oil of the nigella sativa seed, also called blackseed or black cumin seed, among other names. A tablespoon per day is taken on an empty stomach. It fights h. pylori and yeast and is gastro-protective.

It is not recommended for women (or men) with high estrogen (estrogen dominance). It also has a strong taste and may be best consumed in capsule form.

GARLIC:

Not everyone can tolerate garlic due to intolerance, reflux triggers or bacterial overgrowth, but it has powerful anti h. pylori activity. The active antibacterial ingredient in garlic is called allicin. You can take allicin in supplement form. Allicin does not typically trigger symptoms in people who react to garlic. This is my favorite brand of Allicin. Take one to 3 capsules daily with food.

PROPOLIS:

Propolis is made by honey bees to hold their hives together. Propolis extract, available in supplement form, can inhibit the growth of h. pylori bacteria due to high content of phenolic compounds. It also supports the immune system.

DIE OFF REACTION

You may find that things get worse before getting better. This is due to the die off reaction.

As pathogens die off they release endotoxins. Endotoxic die off can clog and overwhelm detox channels and drainage pathways and cause flu-like symptoms, new symptoms or the worsening of old or current symptoms.

This reaction can be remedied by opening drainage and detox pathways or cutting down on/taking a break from supplements until the reaction passes.

Here are a few ways to open detox/drainage pathways in the liver, kidneys, and bowels:

Drink more water

Take epsom salt baths

Sweat in a sauna

Castor oil packs

Move lymphatic fluid with massage,

skin dry brushing or jumping on a trampoline (rebounding)

If your bowels get sluggish take magnesium citrate to move them.

Since coconut oil is highly antibacterial, oil pulling, or swishing a tablespoon of coconut oil in the mouth for 20 minutes, can help detox the mouth, which can help detox the gut (we swallow the bacteria in the mouth).

Also, h. pylori can live in the oral cavity and oil pulling is a great way to detox it as part of a morning routine. You may want to change toothbrushes after you complete your protocol.

Typically h. pylori protocols are well tolerated compared to other pathogen-killing protocols, but prioritize rest and give your body what it needs during this time.

WHEN WILL I FEEL BETTER?

"When will I feel better?" is one of the most common questions I am asked by clients. There's no universal answer. Everyone is different and you may feel worse before you feel better.

While feeling better is encouraging, not feeling better doesn't mean that progress is not happening. The body repairs slowly, so be patient and don't let anxiety slow you down further.

Sometimes people don't start feeling better until their stomach acid bounces back. It takes a bit of time for the stomach's parietal cells to repair after the protocol ends.

Also, if you have other gut infections, you may not feel better until you clear those too.

Stay consistent, know you're doing your best and trust your body to heal.

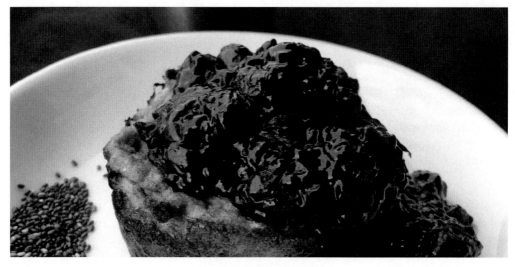

SUPPORTIVE HERBS AND FOODS

The following foods help eradicate h. pylori and make your protocol more successful.

Each food has a special role in debilitating and weakening h. pylori bacteria in a unique way, thus lowering it's defenses.

CRANBERRY JUICE:

Cranberry juice prevents h. pylori from sticking to the stomach walls where it lives. Without the protection of the mucosal barrier it becomes more vulnerable to eradication.

It is important to consume unsweetened cranberry juice. You don't need a lot of cranberry juice for this to be effective. A few ounces a day is all you need. Taking it on an empty stomach works best but if that's irritating take it with food.

BROCCOLI SPROUTS:

You can consume fresh broccoli sprouts or use the supplement form. Fresh sprouts are easy to grow. I provide growing instructions at the end of this guide.

It's more concentrated in supplement form and does not require growing fresh sprouts. Supplements may be the easiest option, and 2 capsules a day is all you need.

Broccoli sprouts help inhibit an enzyme that allows h. pylori to move freely through the mucosal barrier and escape eradication.

Broccoli sprouts also contain sulforaphane which was shown to kill h. pylori in mouse studies.

GREEN TEA/MATCHA:

Green tea helps inhibit the function of efflux pumps that can spit out the antibiotics or antimicrobials used to kill h. pylori. One cup of green tea a day can do this.

Efflux pumps are transport proteins involved in the extrusion of toxic substances (including antibiotics) from the cells. They are found in gram negative and gram positive bacteria to protect against antibiotics and may be responsible for antibiotic resistance in some cases.

Any type of green tea is effective in disarming these pumps. If you are sensitive to caffeine you can choose decaffeinated green tea. Green tea also decreases h. pylori activity and is anti inflammatory.

A 2009 study on mice showed that green tea slowed h. pylori growth. Consuming green tea before an onset of infection lowers the severity of stomach inflammation. Consuming the tea during an infection reduces the severity of gastritis.

PREVENTING RELAPSE OR REINFECTION

It is true that h. pylori can come back. Knowing this is disturbing. But worrying about this before clearing the infection is very counterproductive, stressful and discouraging.

Stress raises your chances of reinfection or reactivation, creating a self-fulfilling prophecy.

Worrying about reinfection is a trauma response. Once you understand how to spot it, test for it and treat it, it won't cause the same level of problems. By addressing it immediately you'll head off the downstream problems it can cause.

If h. pylori does come back and begins to cause problems again, you now know how to get rid of it. Simply keep calm and treat again.

Here are some strategies to help lower chances of reinfection significantly:

Retest to make sure h. pylori is g one.

If you used the GI Map to initially test for it, I suggest retesting with that. Diagnostic Solutions has a less expensive h. pylori only test.

You must wait at least 6 weeks after stopping the h. pylori herbs to retest.

Sometimes people will feel better after the first round of herbs because the infection has diminished but not gone away completely. If so, it can grow back with stress or immune suppression.

One more round of herbs will do the trick.

It is very important to retest to make sure it's truly gone, and to prevent chances of regrowth.

Also, test family members and don't share drinking glasses or utensils with them until they are tested

H. pylori is easily passed back and forth by family members. Test everyone in your household or family members you have close contact with. Even the dog.

Treating everyone who tests positive is the best way to prevent reinfection.

Support your adrenals and diffuse stress when it hits

Self care is the best way to prevent stress-induced recurrence.

Get rest, balance blood sugar and take adaptogenic herbs like ashwagandha, tulsi and rhodiola to support adrenals.

A strong immune system and well functioning adrenals are powerful defenses against recurrence.

Taking Saccharomyces Boulardii will help support your immune system.

Supplement with broccoli sprouts, propolis or black seed oil if things begin to feel off.

Minimize self reinfection

After you finish your treatment protocol it is a good idea to swap out your toothbrushes or soak them in Matula tea, get rid of lipstick or chapstick and disinfect night guards in white vinegar.

Anything that comes in contact with your mouth or saliva should be cleaned or thrown out to minimize chances of reinfection. And because h. pylori can live in the mouth and dental plaque, getting your teeth cleaned immediately after you finish your protocol could prevent chances of dental reinfection.

PROBIOTICS AND H. PYLORI

Probiotics secrete antibacterial substances such as lactic acid, short chain fatty acids, hydrogen peroxide and bacteriocins to lower numbers of spiral bacteria, like h. pylori.

Also, some probiotic strains help increase mucin production to protect the gastric mucosal barrier against the adherence of pathogenic bacteria such as h. pylori.

Probiotics have also been shown to increase the success rates of antibiotic and herbal treatments for h. pylori and reduce the damage done by antibiotics.

There's one probiotic that's particularly helpful and has been well studied.

Saccharomyces boulardii (Sac B) is the most helpful probiotic for h. pylori. It's technically a yeast that exhibits powerful probiotic properties. It has very strong immune supporting and modulating properties. It is also ok to take with bacterial overgrowth in the small intestine or if you react to regular probiotics.

Sac B also flushes out bacterial overgrowth of the clostridia species, that often accompanies h. pylori. Clostridia can increase the stress response, cause sleep issues and prevent people from truly and deeply relaxing. Not only does it help the biome recover from antibiotics use, but it will help prevent yeast overgrowth due to antibiotics.

For those with yeast and bacterial overgrowth, I also recommend a spore-based probiotic called Megasporbiotic. It supports the immune system and biome and has strong antimicrobial properties (it kills the bad guys).

This is a powerful probiotic that needs to be started slowly (open the capsule and start with ¼ to ½ daily) You can find it in Amazon. Search for it after creating an account. I don't suggest buying supplements on Amazon due to the rampant amount of counterfeit herbs.

Lactobacillus reuteri is another probiotic option for supporting the health of the delicate stomach lining. It is available in a supplement called Gatro-ease by Life eExtension, which also contains zinc carnosine.

HOW TO EAT FOR H. PYLORI

How you eat can be as important as what you eat.

Here are strategies to boost digestion and minimize undigested food particles that feed bacterial and yeast overgrowth in the small intestine.

Don't eat while stressed

Eating while stressed will reduce stomach acid even further. Before you eat, do some deep belly breathing to calm your system and get it ready for digestion. Three deep breaths and a longer exhale will move your system into a rest and digest state.

Cook your foods well

Low stomach acid makes it harder to digest foods like raw veggies, meat, fatty foods, and complex grains (simple grains like white rice are easier to break down than oatmeal and quinoa). Cook veggies well. Slow cook, pressure cook or stew your meat until it breaks apart with a fork.

Soak, puree or blend your food

The easiest foods to digest have been broken down through cooking methods like pressure cooking, slow cooking, blending, stewing or pureeing.

Soaking hard- to-digest foods like nuts or beans before cooking or consuming them will boost digestibility and be easier on the gut lining by breaking down harmful lectins and phytic acid, which can irritate and damage the gut lining.

Eat smaller and more frequent meals

You may notice that your symptoms are worse on an empty stomach. But overfilling your stomach can also trigger symptoms.

Don't leave the tank too empty or overfill it.

Eating too much overwhelms the stomach's ability to digest. Some people with h. pylori feel better when they eat smaller and more frequent meals.

These dietary changes and frequency are temporary to support gut repair. You will most likely be able to return to eating salads with raw veggies and bigger, fatty meats after stomach acid production returns.

Strong digestion will help you tolerate more foods and protect you better against contaminated foods/ food poisoning.

WHAT TO EAT FOR H. PYLORI

Generally a healthy, whole food diet will lower inflammation, balance the biome and support immunity, which will help the gut heal. Try to minimize processed food and eat your veggies.

During an h. pylori protocol, there are only a few inflammatory foods that are important to avoid such as coffee, gluten, dairy, alcohol and refined sugar.

For some people, goat and sheep dairy may be a good swap for cow dairy because it is easier to digest and better tolerated.

Coffee in particular can thin and irritate an already inflamed and raw stomach lining and increase chances of pain and ulcer.

Coffee is hard to give up, so I suggest swapping it for a hot morning drink like matcha or regular green tea. Green tea does double duty of providing a caffeine fix and helping fight h. pylori.

There are a few foods to emphasize for h. pylori eradication and support.

Some of which soothe the stomach lining, while others have targeted antimicrobial activity.

Broccoli sprouts are probably the most powerful foods you can consume for h. pylori and I provided instructions for growing them below. Cabbage juice contains vitamin U, which fights h. pylori and repairs gastritis and ulcers.

Celery juice helps increase gastric acid and lower inflammation.

Here's a complete list:

H. pylori fighting foods

- Cabbage juice (Vitamin U, along with glutamine and methionine in the juice are the active ingredients).

- Celery juice

- Manuka honey (targeted antibacterial activity)

- Coconut oil and coconut meat (coconut flakes, coconut butter and coconut milk)

- Unsweetened cranberry juice

- Olive oil

- Garlic (fresh or roasted)

- Turmeric

- Cinnamon powder

- Fresh broccoli sprouts and broccoli

- Organic berries

I've included 11 healthy recipes at the end of this guide, that use some of these foods to fight h. pylori deliciously.

HOW TO GROW BROCCOLI SPROUTS

Broccoli sprouts kill and debilitate h. pylori, kill viruses, detox the liver and protect against cancer.

Broccoli sprouts are whole broccoli plants that are only 4 days old. They are considered a low FODMAP food. Their active ingredient is sulforaphane.

They are the "SUPEREST" of superfoods and inexpensive to grow. Add them to pesto, blend them into a smoothie or add them to a wrap or salad.

You can also buy fresh broccoli sprouts at the supermarket.

Here's my recipe for an h. pylori super shake using a tray of sprouts and other h. pylori fighting foods.

H. PYLORI SUPERSHAKE

Blend ½ to 1 tray of fresh broccoli sprouts (4 days old) with ½ a cup of coconut milk and half a banana for sweetness.

Optional add-ins are ½ clove of raw garlic, 1 teaspoon of manuka honey and ½ teaspoon of propolis powder from an open propolis capsule.

HOW TO GROW SPROUTS

Buy organic broccoli seeds and a 4 tray seed sprouter.

I like the 4 tray sprouter because you can start a new batch daily and they take 4 days to grow.

To start the first batch, soak one tablespoon of broccoli seeds in water for 6 to 8 hours.

Transfer the soaked seeds to one of the trays and water one or two times daily with half a cup of water. I find that watering once a day produces the best sprouts but you may have to water more in a drier, hotter climate. The water will drip down to the bottom tray through all the layers and needs to be emptied daily.

Keep adding a new tray daily to the stack and watering as instructed.

Keep the tray out of direct sunlight. And don't worry if a white fuzz starts to grow. That is not mold, just part of the broccoli plant.

After 4 days, the first tray is ready to be consumed.

Consume one tray daily and make sure to start another tray once you have emptied one, to keep the process going.

It's that easy.

If you have questions about how to grow sprouts or anything else reach out to me at angelaprivin@yahoo.com

Meanwhile, enjoy the healing recipes below.

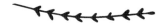

11 RECIPES FOR H. PYLORI

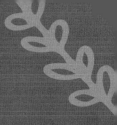

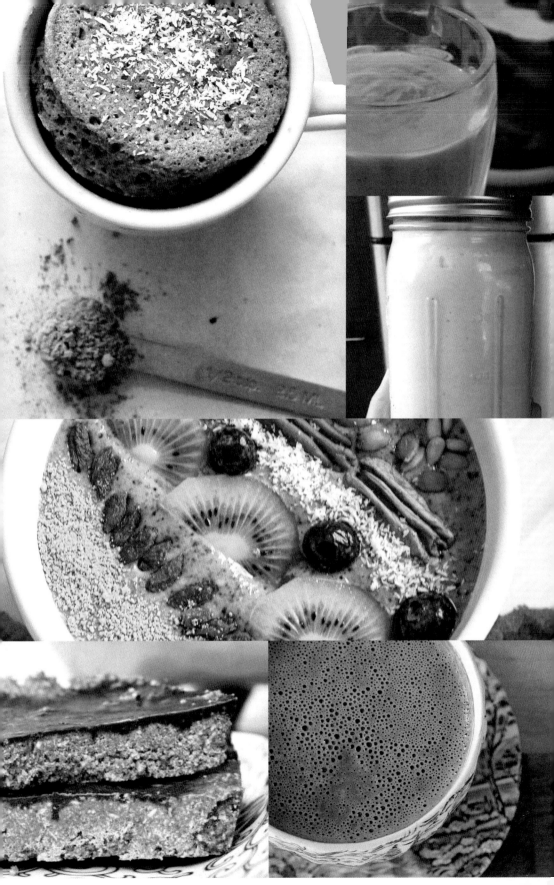

H. PYLORI MATCHA
Mug Cake

(ACTIVE INGREDIENT MATCHA GREEN TEA AND MANUKA HONEY)

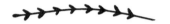

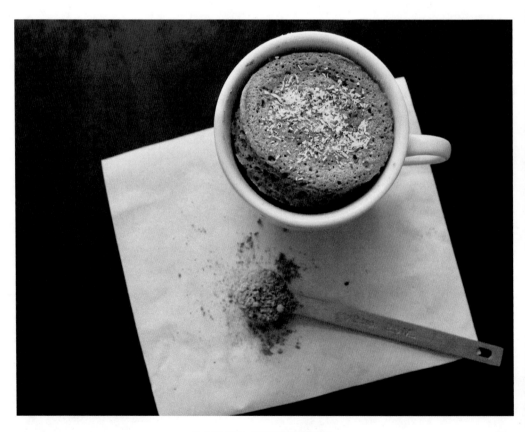

Enjoy this green-tea flavored mug cake for a quick, convenient and portion-controlled treat that helps fight h. pylori. Both green tea and manuka honey have active anti-h. pylori ingredients. This recipe takes under 5 minutes to make and includes an egg-free version. Enjoy with a matcha golden milk latte.

Ingredients

4 Tablespoons of nut or seed flour

½ to 1 teaspoon of matcha green tea powder (depending on how strong you like it)

¼ teaspoon of baking powder

1 Tablespoon of raw local honey (Manuka is best for h. Pylori)

3 Tablespoons of non-dairy milk (I used coconut milk)

½ teaspoon of vanilla powder or extract

1 egg

1 tablespoon of melted coconut oil

Optional: 1-2 Tablespoons of dried cranberries

Optional: 1 teaspoon of collagen

Egg free version

½ teaspoon to 1 teaspoon of matcha

4 Tablespoons of non-dairy milk

½ teaspoon of vanilla powder or extract

Pinch of salt

1 Tablespoon of honey (I used Manuka)

¼ teaspoon of baking soda

1 teaspoon of melted coconut oil (avocado oil or melted butter can also work)

2 Tablespoons of cassava flour

How to

Mix ingredients together in a mug.

Every microwave is different and will take between 60 and 90 second to "bake". The mug cake will start to rise and should be done after 90 seconds. If not fully cooked, microwave for 15 second increments until done. The dough will rise as it cooks so don't overfill your mug.

If using the oven method, preheat your oven to 350 and bake for 15 to 20 minutes with the dough divided between two silicon muffin tins or oven safe ramekins.

CRANBERRY
Jelly

(ACTIVE INGREDIENT CRANBERRY)

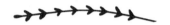

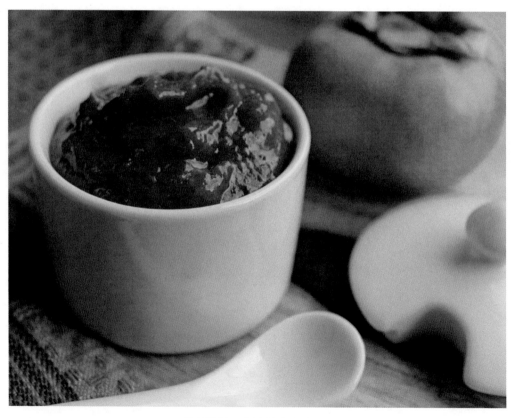

Cranberry is a powerful h. pylori-fighting food. Here's a recipe for homemade cranberry jelly that's lower in sugar than store bought jelly and contains collagen, which rebuilds the lining of the stomach. A delicious way to reduce h. pylori overgrowth.

Ingredients

1 cup of organic, fresh cranberries

1 persimmon, peeled and cut into
8 pieces
(can sub apple or pear)

2 dates

Juice of ½ a lime or lemon

1 teaspoon of gelatin

Optional: 2 Tablespoons of tart
cherry juice
(can use unsweetened cranberry
juice or pomegranate
juice instead)

How to

Boil the cranberries in water for 10 minutes. They will make popping noises as they boil. Don't stand too close to the pot so you don't get splashed as they pop.

Soak the dates in a bowl of hot water for 10 minutes to soften.

Drain the cranberries and put them in a food processor or powerful blender with the diced persimmon, dates, lime juice and cherry juice, if using.

Process the mixture until you get a smooth puree. Add a teaspoon of gelatin and process for another minute until thoroughly mixed in.

Transfer the mixture to a covered dish and leave in the fridge for a few hours for the jelly to set.

Note: If you would like a firmer jelly, double the amount of gelatin

PESTO
With Garlic Oil

(ACTIVE INGREDIENT BROCCOLI SPROUTS AND OLIVE OIL)

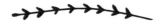

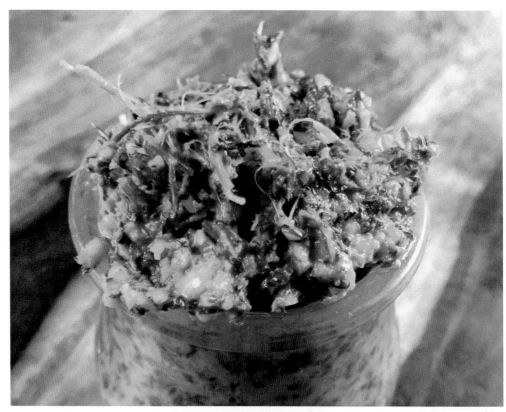

Another easy way to add broccoli sprouts to your meal is in homemade pesto. The herbs in this pesto help with liver detox and olive oil has active anti-h. pylori activity.

Start with a handful of broccoli sprouts and increase according to your taste and tolerance. Slowly work up to 1 cup of broccoli sprouts and 1 cup of other herbs for an extremely medicinal pesto to top salads, fish and roasted veggies.

Ingredients

½ cup of pumpkin seeds or other nuts

2 cups of green herbs: can use a mix of broccoli sprouts, cilantro, basil and/or parsley.
¼ cup of garlic olive oil or regular olive oil (use more if you want a thinner pesto)

1-2 fresh garlic cloves, minced

¼ teaspoon of salt

Juice of ½ a lemon

Broccoli sprouts

Optional: if you can't tolerate garlic add ¼ teaspoon of hing (asafoetida)

How to make pesto

Put all the ingredients, including the optional ones, in a blender or food processor and blend.

If you want the pesto to be thinner, add more oil.

How to make garlic oil

Garlic oil is OK to consume on a low FODMAP or GERD diet because the fructan content does not leach into the oil, while the flavor does. The more garlic you add to the oil, the stronger the garlic flavor will be.

I added 2 cloves of chopped garlic per ½ cup of oil for a stronger garlic taste.

The oil should be refrigerated and used within 3 to 4 days. You can safely freeze the oil for as long as you want.

Olive oil will solidify and turn cloudy in the fridge but is fine to use.

How to make pesto

Put all the ingredients, including the optional ones, in a blender or food processor and blend.

if you want the pesto to be thinner, add more oil.

COCONUT BREAKFAST
Bites /Bars

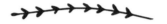

(ACTIVE INGREDIENT TURMERIC, COCONUT AND CINNAMON)

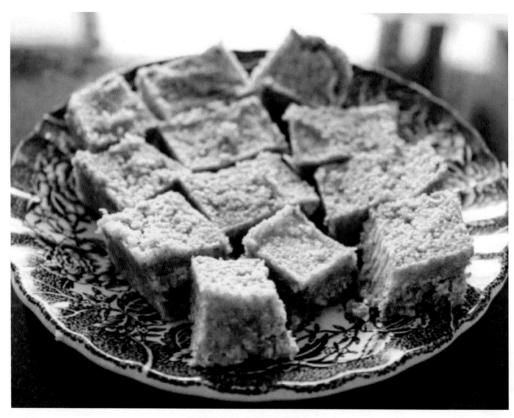

This no-bake treat is full of shredded coconut and coconut oil to fight h. pylori. I eat it for breakfast because it doesn't spike blood sugar, while being lightly sweet and full of good fats and protein. I've included two flavor variations and this treat lends itself to improvisation. You can add whatever nuts, seeds, spices, dried fruit, nut butter or sweeteners you have on hand. It needs to be chilled in the fridge and will start to soften and melt above 78 degrees.

Ingredients

1 cup of shredded coconut

1 Tablespoon of nut butter or melted coconut butter (or both)

1 Tablespoon of sweetener (I used honey but maple syrup also works)

⅓ cup (5 to 6 tablespoons) of melted coconut oil

Matcha flavor

½-1 teaspoon of matcha (depending on how strong you like it)

½ teaspoon of vanilla powder or extract

Optional: For a creamy latte flavor, add
1 Tablespoon of coconut cream

Golden milk latte version

½ teaspoon of vanilla powder or extract

½ teaspoon of cinnamon

½ teaspoon of cardamom

½ teaspoon of powdered ginger

¼ to ½ teaspoon of turmeric

Pinch of black pepper

Optional: for a creamier latte flavor, add 1 Tablespoon of coconut cream

How to

Melt coconut oil by submerging glass bottle in hot water. If your coconut oil comes in a plastic bottle, transfer it to a heat-safe container before melting.

Combine all the ingredients and mix well. You can mix the ingredients in a bowl and then transfer to container. I used a small silicone bread loaf pan to set the bars and mixed all the ingredients directly inside of it with a fork.

Once everything is well mixed, put in the fridge for 1 hour to set.
Slice into bars or squares and serve.

These will start to melt if kept above room temperature for too long. It's best to store them in the fridge where they should keep for a long time if you're not adding fresh berries. But they never last long in my house because they're too good.

MATCHA GOLDEN
Milk Latte

(ACTIVE INGREDIENT GREEN TEA, COCONUT, TURMERIC AND CINNAMON)

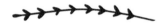

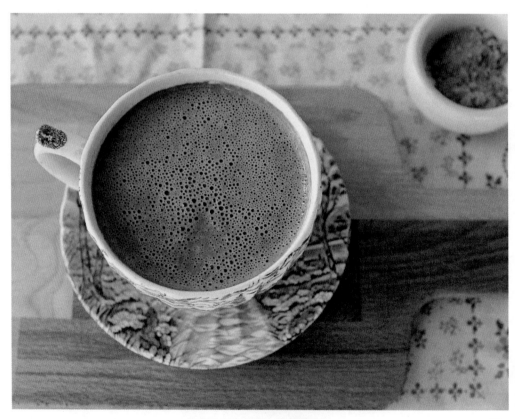

Golden milk is a popular, anti-inflammatory, hot drink full of turmeric, ginger, cinnamon and other healing spices. It has been used medicinally in the Ayurvedic tradition from India. I've added matcha green tea powder to this ancient drink. If you don't have any matcha powder you can steep a green tea bag in a cup of hot water.

Ingredients

1 teaspoon of coconut oil

¾ teaspoon of matcha powder

1 cup of hot water

1 cup of non dairy milk (coconut, nut or seed milk)

¼ teaspoon of ginger

¼ teaspoon of cardamom

¼ teaspoon of cinnamon

¼ teaspoon of vanilla

½ teaspoon of turmeric

Pinch of black pepper

Honey to taste

Optional: 1 teaspoon of collagen powder

How to

Heat the water and the non dairy milk together in a pan.

Mix in coconut oil, spices and matcha powder.

This drink tastes best blended. If you leave it for too long after blending, it may taste slightly gritty. Blend or mix again before enjoying.

FLAVORED COCONUT
Butter Cups

(ACTIVE INGREDIENT COCONUT BUTTER)

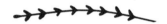

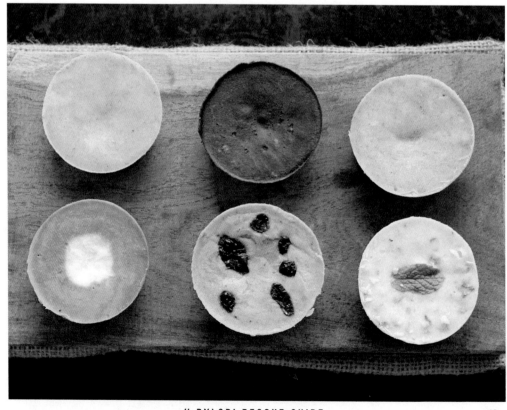

Coconut butter is a low-sugar snack full of healthy fats and is an immune-boosting antimicrobial food. You can eat coconut butter out of the jar, but I make them into snack-sized bon bons with added flavorings for fun and variety. The matcha green tea, golden milk and chai spice flavorings are particularly good for h. pylori. Avoid the mint flavor if you have reflux. These are best kept in temperatures below 78 degrees f.

You can toast coconut butter to bring out its sweetness. Get the recipe for my toasted coconut butter cups in my Treats That Heal cookbook.

Ingredients

1 cup of coconut butter, melted

Optional flavor mix ins: (choose one of the following or mix and match)

Matcha green tea latte: ½ teaspoon of matcha powder, or more if you like a stronger flavor

Nut butter and jelly: ¼ cup of nut butter and ¼ cup of chopped, dried fruit of choice

Mint: 1 to 2 tablespoons of freshly chopped mint or ½ teaspoon of mint extract

Carob: ¼ cup of carob powder (can sub cocoa powder and add a tablespoon of honey and ¼ teaspoon of vanilla extract or powder)

Chai spice: ½ teaspoon each of cinnamon, cardamom, ginger, vanilla (chai spice)

Golden milk latte: Add ¼ teaspoon of turmeric and a pinch of black pepper to the chai spices above

Note: other options I have not tried personally but would be delicious:

Lemonade: ½ teaspoon of lemon zest and the juice of ½ lemon juice with a teaspoon of honey

Maple dream: Tablespoon of maple syrup with ½ teaspoon of pumpkin spice

Marzipan: 1 teaspoon of amaretto extract and chopped almonds

Or try your own favorite flavors or mix ins....

How to

Melt the coconut butter in a microwave, sauce pan or submerge the whole glass jar in hot water until it softens into a pourable texture.

Stir the suggested flavorings into one cup of coconut butter and mix well. Or improvise with your own flavorings.

Pour into candy molds or muffin tins (regular or mini) and chill in the fridge for one hour.

If you want to make multiple flavors, divide the coconut butter into 3rds and divide each flavoring ingredient by a third and mix in. Store in an airtight container in the fridge if your kitchen is above 70 degrees or on the kitchen counter if the room temp is below 70 degrees.

POLYPHENOL
Berry Jam

(ACTIVE INGREDIENT BERRIES)

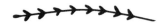

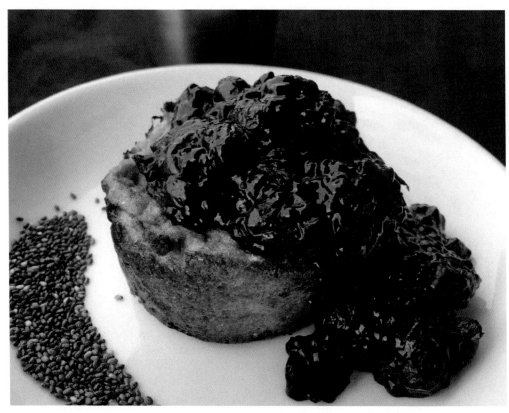

Polyphenols feed keystone bacterial strains in your large intestine, which support immunity. Immune function is key to clearing h. pylori. Berries also fight h. pylori directly. This jam can also be made with cranberries (add an extra tablespoon of sweetener). This jam also contains fiber from chia seeds, which encourages faster gastric emptying.

Ingredients

4 cups of berries, frozen or fresh
(I used frozen blueberries only,
but you can add sweeter fruit like
chopped papaya, pineapple or
mango)

2 tablespoons of coconut water

1 tablespoon of lemon juice

¼ cup of chia seeds

Optional: 1 teaspoon of manuka
honey or maple syrup

How to

In a bowl, mix blueberries with lemon juice and coconut water and muddle it with a fork to release the juice.

In a saucepan, cook the fruit on medium heat for about 15 minutes to bring out its natural sugars. Stir while you cook to keep the mixture from burning.

Let cool for 20 minutes.

Add chia seeds and mix well.

Put in the fridge overnight.

Taste and adjust sweetness with extra honey.

Store in the fridge in an airtight container for up to 4 or 5 days.

BROCCOLI SPROUT GREEN
Smoothie Bowl

(ACTIVE INGREDIENT BROCCOLI SPROUTS, BERRIES AND BONE BROTH)

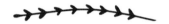

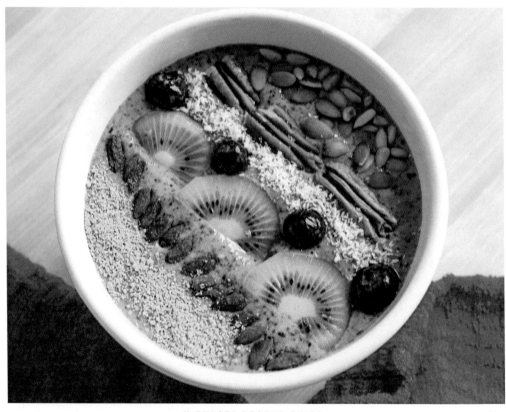

Green smoothies are a great way to enjoy broccoli sprouts and leafy greens, which could otherwise be hard to digest. Blending breaks down the vegetable fiber making it easier to break down and assimilate. Adding sweet ingredients to smoothies such as fruit covers up the taste of the greens and sprouts. Berries fight h. pylori and bananas are soothing to the stomach and gut. Bone broth is an extremely healing food that helps repair the lining of the stomach and intestine. The fruit and nut milk/coconut water can also disguises the taste of the broth.

Ingredients

1 ripe banana (sliced, fresh or frozen)

½ to 1 cup of bone broth (fat strained)

¼ cup of fresh or frozen berries

1 cup of coconut water, nut milk, water OR coconut milk

Greens. Quantity to taste (start with a handful of greens and add more each time)
I use 2 cups of greens. Choose from kale, spinach, arugula, romaine or spring mix.

½ cup of broccoli sprouts

How to make a smoothie bowl

Put all ingredients in a blender and blend well until all the ingredients are combined.

Pour in a bowl and decorate with

Bee Pollen
Berries
Pumpkin seeds or pecans
Shredded coconut
Nut butter
Melted coconut butter
Cocoa nibs
Spirulina powder
Chia and/or flax seeds
Sliced bananas
Dried cranberries

How to

Add all ingredients and blend well. Taste as you go.

YOUNG COCONUT
Yogurt

(ACTIVE INGREDIENT COCONUT AND PROBIOTICS)

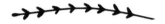

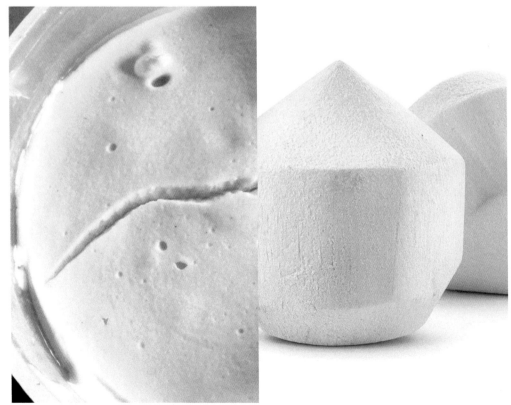

Coconut is an antimicrobial food that fights bacteria (like h. pylori), yeast and viruses, while probiotics support the biome and immune system. This coconut yogurt is delicious, clean and easy to make. All you need is a young coconut, probiotic capsule and blender. A yogurt maker makes it easier but you can also make this in an oven. Young coconuts have an ivory shell and are sold online, at Asian grocery stores or specialty supermarkets.

Ingredients

3 young coconuts (all the young coconut meat scraped from the inside and the coconut water inside).

One serving of your favorite probiotic capsule or powder or two tablespoons of yogurt from an unsweetened, unflavored yogurt.

All probiotic capsules are opened up and only the powder is used.

Make sure the probiotic contains the appropriate strains for making yogurt which includes a few of these strains: lactobacillus acidophilus, bifidobacterium bifidum, bifidobacterium lactis and streptococcus thermophilus.

How to

Open the coconuts by cutting a small hole on top. Easiest way is with a coco jack or use a machete or sharp knife to chop a round or square opening on top. Be careful not to spill the coconut water while opening.

Pour out the coconut water into a container of choice.

Scrape out all the coconut meat using a spoon.

Put the coconut meat in the blender and pour in about 1/4 cup of coconut water and blend. Keep adding coconut water until the coconut meat forms a thick applesauce-like consistency.

Add in the probiotic powder and blend for 30 seconds. Or add in a few tablespoons of unflavored, unsweetened yogurt and blend for 30 seconds.

Pour the contents of the blender into a yogurt maker and turn it on for 12 to 24 hours depending on how strong and sour you like your yogurt to taste. The longer you keep it the higher the probiotic content.

If you don't have a yogurt maker, dehydrator or instant pot, look up directions on how to make yogurt in the oven. I've never personally done it so I can't speak from experience but people do make yogurt this way.

PAPAYA
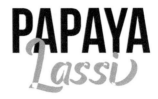
Lassi

(ACTIVE AND SOOTHING INGREDIENTS YOGURT, BANANA AND PAPAYA)

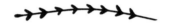

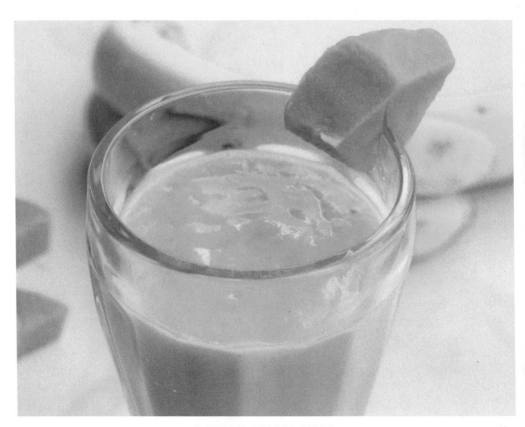

A lassi is a traditional Indian drink that combines yogurt, fruit (mango) and sugar. This lassi is made with papaya, a low sugar fruit that contains natural enzymes that help with digestion. While this lassi won't kill h. pylori bacteria directly, the probiotics from the yogurt plus the soothing, easy to digest fiber from fruit will help create a healing environment in the stomach. This shake is easy to digest and absorb despite low stomach acid.

Ingredients

1 cup of papaya

1 cup of coconut yogurt

½ cup of nut milk or coconut milk (you can use coconut water in a pinch)

¼ teaspoon of cardamom

¼ teaspoon of vanilla extract or ½ teaspoon of vanilla powder

Optional: For extra sweetness, add a half or whole banana (freeze the banana first to create a frothy, milkshake-like texture)

How to

Cut the papaya, remove the seeds and skin.

Put the papaya in a blender with all other ingredients.

Blend well and enjoy.

Note: Papaya seeds have a very powerful anti-parasitic effect. You can add a ½ teaspoon of papaya seeds to this smoothie to give the lassi more medicinal value. The seeds have a strong peppery taste and will change the flavor.

GINGER
Pickle

(ACTIVE INGREDIENT GINGER)

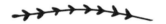

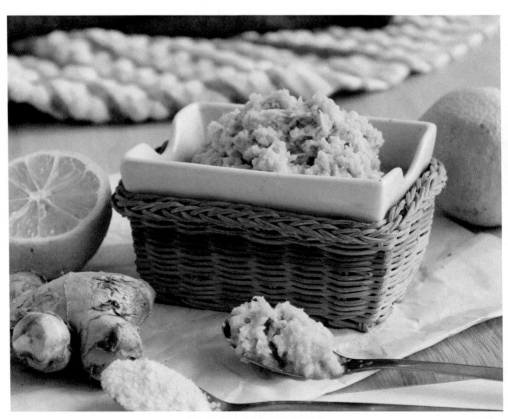

Ginger pickle comes from Indian traditional medicine, and is used as a digestive aid. The salt and lemon preserves the ginger so it can last in your fridge for up to a week, and possibly longer.

Ginger is a powerful antioxidant and anti-inflammatory food that naturally fights infections and helps stimulate digestion and motility. It also helps food leave the stomach quicker.

In Japanese cuisine, sliced pickled ginger is served alongside sushi, as a natural antimicrobial agent that protects against parasites and other pathogens found in raw fish.

Ginger is also great for easing nausea and chronic indigestion.

Take a small pinch before your meal to support digestion and defend against pathogens.

Ingredients

1 ginger root the size of the palm of your hand, peeled and grated (I used a microplane grater to grate mine.

A cheese grater also works.)

1 lemon, juiced

1 teaspoon of salt

How to

Mix ingredients in a glass jar and leave out overnight to slightly ferment.

Once fermented, store in the fridge.

Take ½ to 1 teaspoon before bigger meals every day for 2 to 4 weeks.

Start with a small pinch to get accustomed to the strong taste.

This has kept in my fridge for weeks. Discard if it starts to grow mold.

WANT MORE GUTFRIENDLY TREATS AND RECIPES?

CHECK OUT MY TREATS THAT HEAL COOKBOOK AT

diyhealthblog.com

H. pylori protocol summary sheet

Primary killing herbs (can do both or either one)

Mastic gum- 3000 milligrams daily, split up into two 500 mg capsules three times a day with meals.

Matula tea- Two teabags a day on an empty stomach (90 minutes before and after food) Can reuse each tea bag once.

This protocol is done for 60 days.

Primary supporting herbs (will improve efficacy of primary herbs)

NAC- Three capsules a day with food, divided between three meals (one per meal). This will bust biofilm.

DGL- ⅛ teaspoon of the powder in a few ounces of water 15 minutes before a meal. Or one capsule/ chewable before each meal. This will heal the stomach lining and kill h. pylori.

Saccharomyces Boulardii- Two a day on an empty stomach (30 minutes before food or 90 minutes after. Do not take with other supplements) This will boost the immune system and support eradication.

Other supplements with anti h. pylori activity

Bismuth

Nigella Sativa/blackseed oil

Garlic in the form of allicin

Propolis

Supporting foods

Broccoli sprouts- 1/2 cup of fresh sprouts a day or use it in capsule form (two capsules a day 30 minutes before a meal)

Cranberry juice- A two to three ounce shot of unsweetened juice

Green tea- One to two cups a day

Cabbage juice for vitamin U and ulcer support- one cup a day

Also enjoy coconut, olive oil, garlic (if tolerated), berries, turmeric and yogurt or fermented foods (if tolerated).

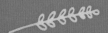